Eat your way to a better relationship

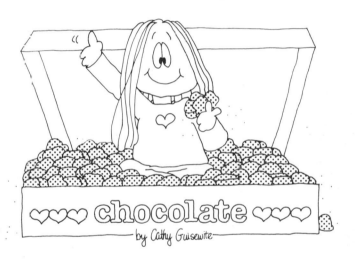

chocolate

by Cathy Guisewite

Andrews and McMeel, Inc.
A Universal Press Syndicate Company

Kansas City ● New York

To Mary Anne

ISBN: 0-8362-1987-2

Library of Congress Catalog Card Number: 82-72420

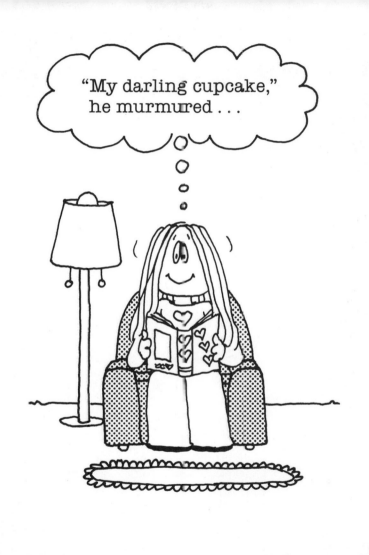

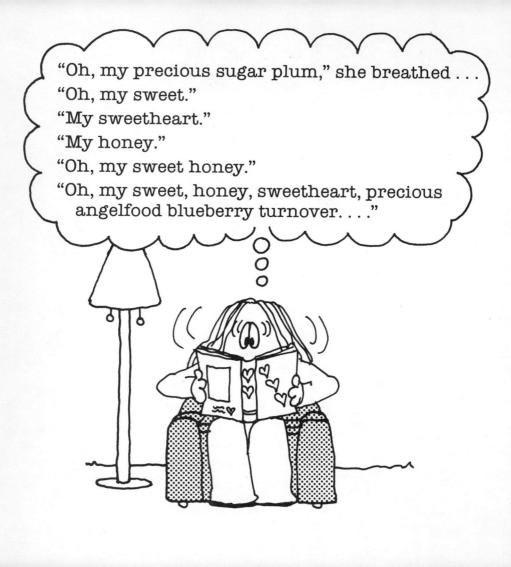

The reader slammed down the book, lunged for the refrigerator, and crammed the "thaw-20-minutes-before-serving" Chocolate-Cheesecake-for-Six directly into her mouth.

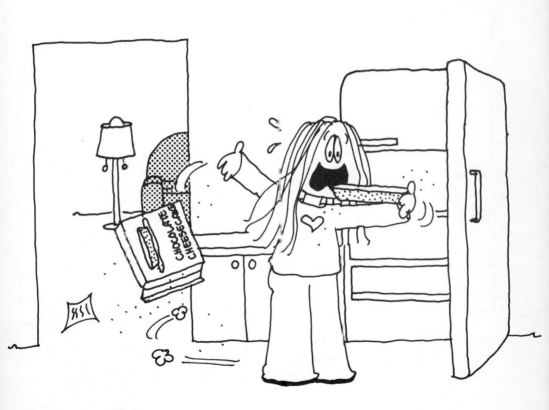

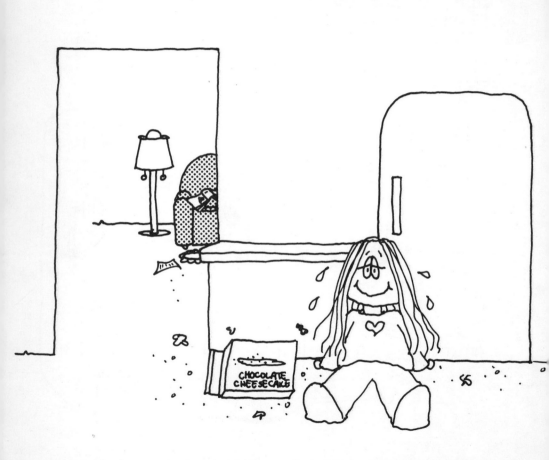

And my mother wonders why we get fat.

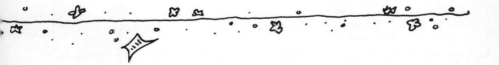

The same woman who whipped up four dozen hot, gooey chocolate chip cookies to help take my mind off the fact that the cute blond in the front row didn't say "hi" to me in the third grade.

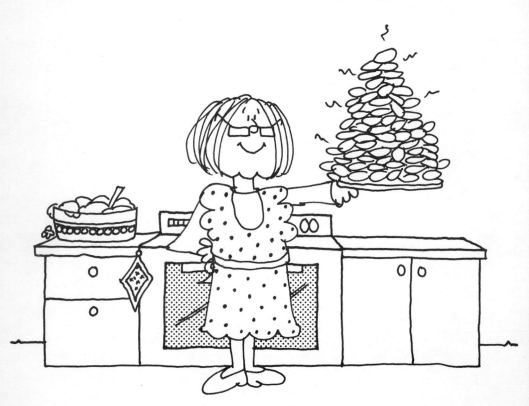

The same woman who baked fudge layer cakes to make up for the special someone who "lost my phone number" for two months, three weeks, 11 days five hours, and 19 minutes in the summer of 1969.

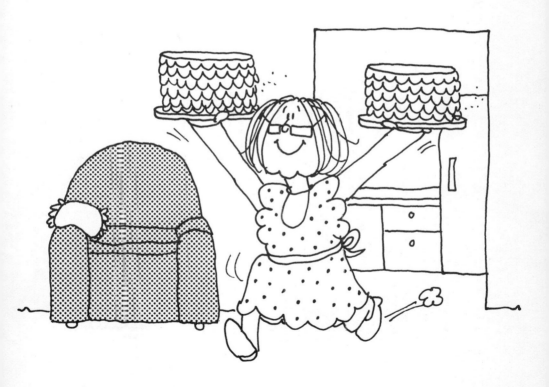

The same woman who said, "Here. Eat this apple pie. You'll forget all about him." (You'll forget all about him because pretty soon you won't be able to fit into anything in your closet and you'll have a whole new set of things to torture yourself about. Mom never mentioned this part.)

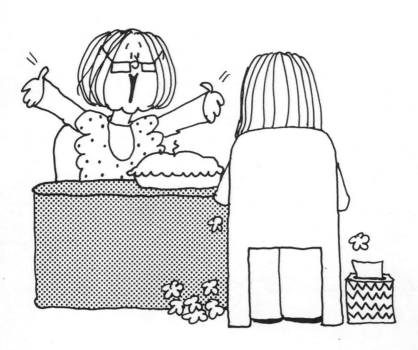

The same woman who was helping me pick out my china pattern before I was even born, just in case I was a girl, would meet some nice young man, fall in love, get married, and have occasion to use it.

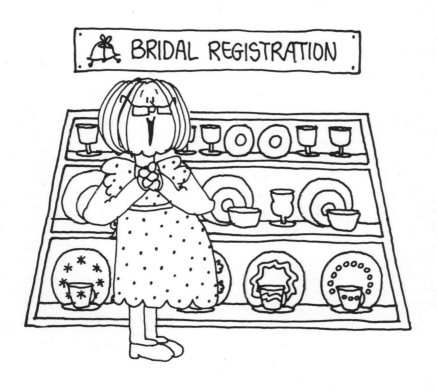

"Think of all the wonderful desserts you could eat off this lovely china," she would say.

"Once you're married and **get** the china, that is."

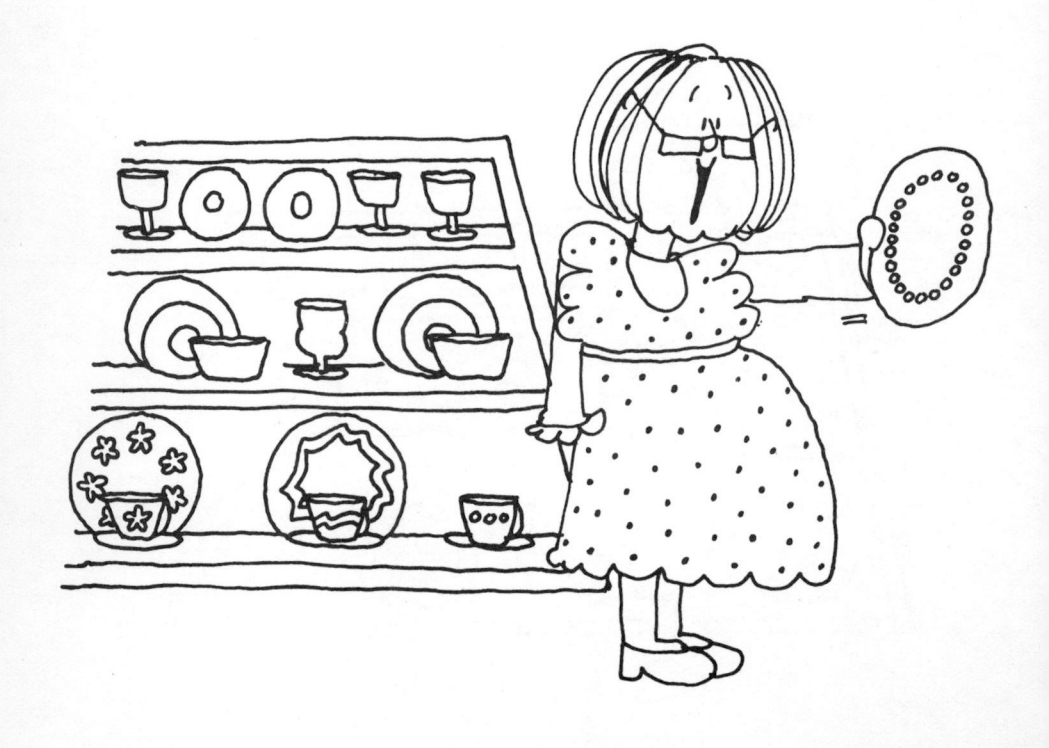

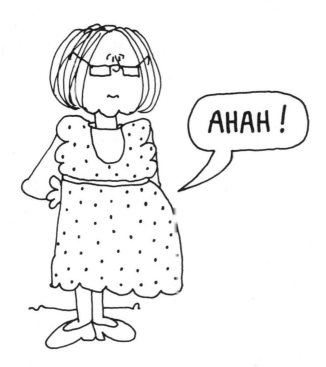

You don't get to eat wonderful desserts off your lovely china until you get your lovely china.

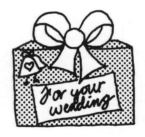

Therefore, get born, meet some nice young man, fall in love, get married, rip open those wedding presents, and look at all the wonderful desserts you'll get to eat off your lovely new china.

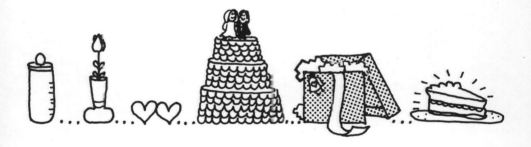

It was all planned out before that first spoonful of Gerber custard pudding even hit my mouth.

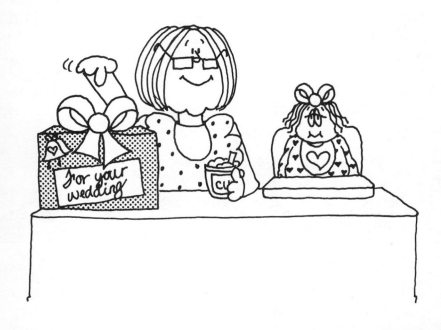

This woman wonders why we get fat.

We know why we get fat, Mother.

We eat.

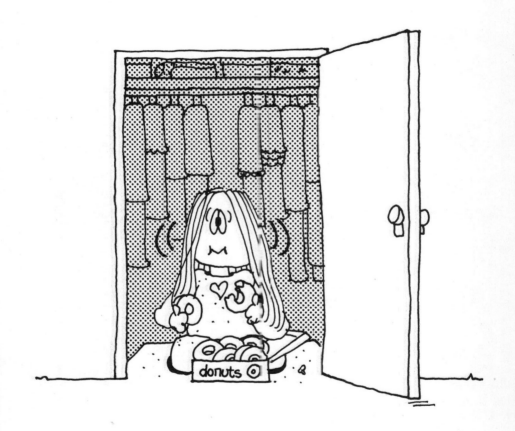

We eat when we're not in love.

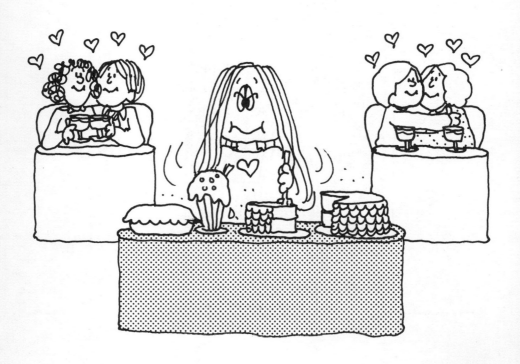

We eat when we want to be in love.

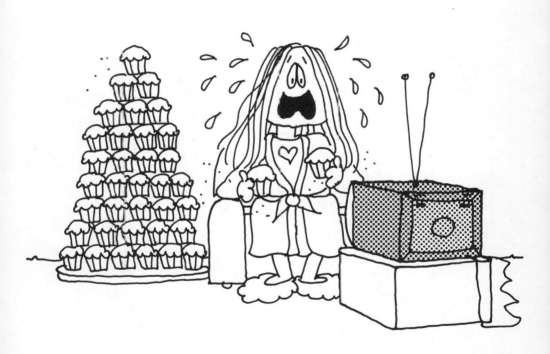

We eat when we don't know whether we're in love or not.

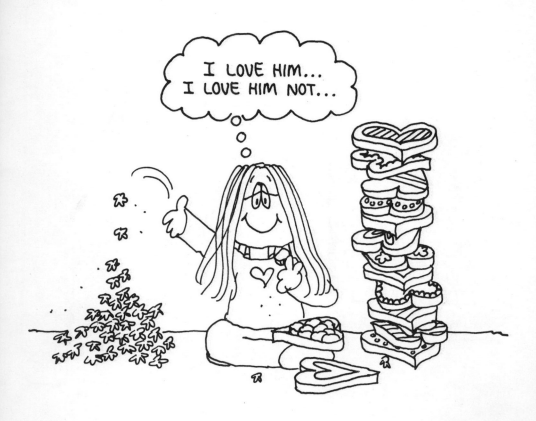

And when we're absolutely positive we're in love, we call each other by fattening food names and expect the thrill of love to magically make the baked Alaska we're plunging into with the new Mr. Right not count.

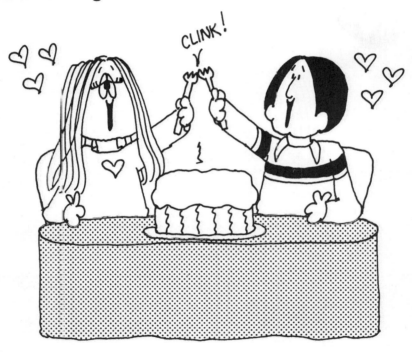

Whoever had a gorgeous man lean over the candlelit table and murmur ...

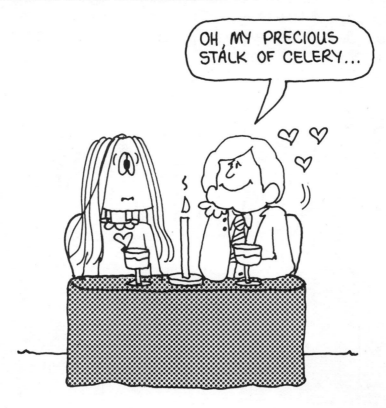

Whoever heard...

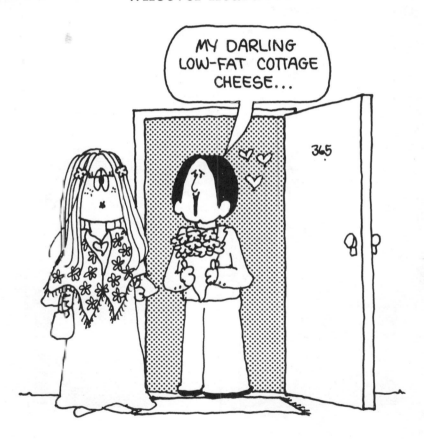

Whoever wanted to stand in the moonlight and be referred to as . . .

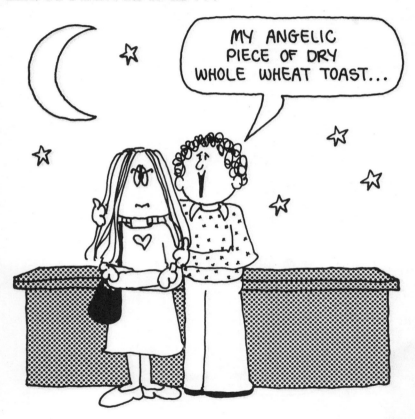

Fattening food and love go together.

Fattening food and love march hand in hand, doughnut

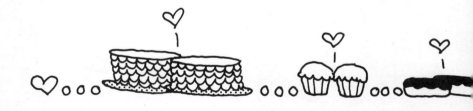

in doughnut, chocolate éclair in chocolate éclair ...

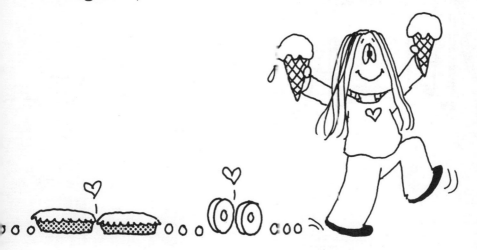

... from the very first moment we noticed that miserable little brat next door had the most ... ahem ... the most delicious blue eyes.

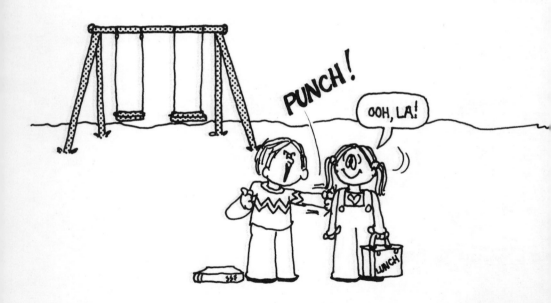

It was okay to overindulge in 1603, when the ideal figure had a 46″ waistline and no one was ever supposed to take enough off for anyone to get a good look at the cellulite.

But it's the '80s.
We have to cope.
We have to quit blaming our stretch
marks on our mothers.
We have to learn to face love without
having a banana split waiting in the wings.

Cases In Point:

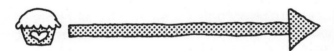

CASE HISTORY #1

On Monday, Oct. 17, 1981, Nora Kramer spotted a boysenberry bismarck in the window of Curtis Pastry Shop on her way to work.

Nora did not buy the boysenberry bismarck, since she was on a strict diet, and had already had seven pieces of sprouted whole wheat toast (fiber) covered with grape jam (two fruit exchanges) for breakfast.

When Nora got to work, she was filled with pride. Then Nora started wishing she was filled with that boysenberry bismarck.

Nora has since eaten at least 300 boysenberry bismarcks, but nothing has even come close to being as perfect and delicious as the one boysenberry bismarck she didn't eat.

A handsome, well-dressed man said "Hi" to Nora one day and Nora opted to not say "Hi" back, since she had just read an article on how to protect yourself from lunatics.

When she got to work, Nora told everyone in the office: "This weirdo said 'Hi' to me, but I had the good sense to not say 'Hi' back."

Nora was self-righteous for about 45 minutes, and then she started wondering. What if the stranger was an optometrist with a place in Malibu? What if the stranger was a famous film maker looking for a new star?

Nora has tried going out with other men. Nora has searched through crowds and made appointments with every optometrist in town.

Nora has dreams about the bismarck she didn't eat. Nora has dreams about the stranger she didn't meet.

Nora is a classic example of the food/love connection.

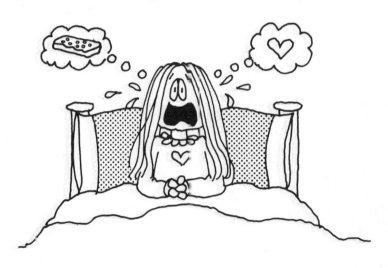

CASE HISTORY #2:

The first thing Jeanette Williams says when you give her something to eat is, "What's in it?"

Even when you give her something totally non-controversial, like an orange, she has to know everything about it.

"Does this have seeds? Where did you get it? What kind of bug spray did the farmers use?"

Serve Jeanette a stuffed flounder with Bordelaise sauce and you can kiss the whole weekend goodbye.

When you first meet Jeanette, you will be totally charmed. Here is a person who finds you so fascinating, she asks questions from the moment you arrive to the moment she says . . .

"Oh, do you have to leave so soon? Why do you have to leave? On your last date what time did you leave? Did she want you to leave, or did you want to leave?

By the end of an evening with Jeanette, you feel like you've been through a food processor. What a coincidence. Try taking Jeanette out to dinner.

Take Jeanette to the Taco Bell, for instance, and you will suddenly be competing with the entire history of the tortilla for her attention.

"Who made this tortilla, and where is he from? Why did he use these particular beans? Is the sauce homemade or trucked in?"

Look closely. The woman you have bared your soul to is now beating her fists on the counter, demanding to know exactly how many grains of salt are added to each individual enchilada and by whom.

Worse, you've made things up to make yourself more interesting to her.

You've bared a soul you don't even have, and you're still on the same level with her as the burrito sauce.

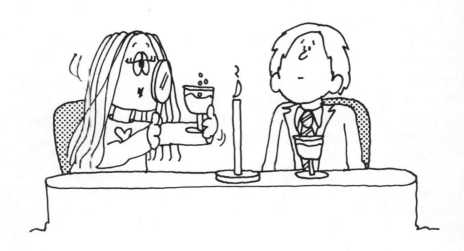

CASE HISTORY #3:

If you want to be friends with Marsha Phillips, you have to be willing to hear what she had for breakfast.

You could be running to an airplane with 19 seconds to make it, screaming with what little breath you have left, "HOLD THE PLANE!! HOLD THE PLANE!!" If Marsha's within earshot, she'll run right up and launch into a 10 minute description of her breakfast.

You could slip on a piece of ice, break your leg in six places, and be writhing in pain while you wait for an ambulance. Marsha will plop down and tell you how she got this stomach ache once from some bad chicken soup.

No matter what you've eaten that's good, Marsha's eaten something better. No matter what you've been poisoned by, Marsha's been closer to death.

No matter what you have going on in your mind, forget it. You're going to hear about Marsha's afternoon snack.

If you have spent time with Marsha and have thought that yours is a private, secretive affair, you should stop and re-think.

Some lady in Arkansas whom you never even met knows the cute thing you said to Marsha at dinner last Tuesday night, when you were wearing that tan tweed sportcoat with the tiny rip on the left cuff.

The entire Walters family, relatives, friends, and pen pals know what flavor breath mint you ate before you kissed Marsha goodnight on Friday.

All of Texas is hoping you don't wear your new brown shoes tomorrow night, since they're sick of hearing about how much Marsha hates them and, frankly, so are all of us here in the Midwest.

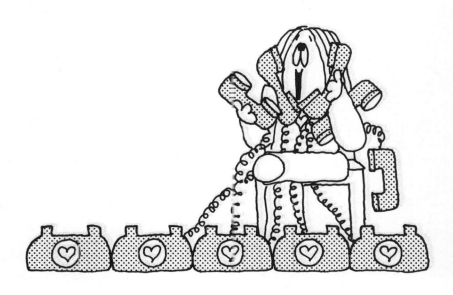

CASE HISTORY #4:

Claire Young was never exactly what you would call a picky eater.

When her grandpa used to take her to Baskin-Robbins 31 Flavors, little Claire would say, "One each."

When tiny, adorable Claire was old enough to read and her parents took her to restaurants, Claire would scan the menu, leap to her feet and demand, "One each!"

Adult Claire isn't even allowed in airport cafeteria lines anymore.

It's not that Claire's a pig. She just doesn't want to miss out on anything.

There were 122 boys in Claire's graduating class in high school. Claire had 122 dates for the senior prom. She finally hid in the bathroom and made her mother deal with all the furious tuxedos at the front door.

It's not that Claire is greedy. She just doesn't want to miss out on anything.

Rumor has it that Claire is packing up her lunch boxes and moving to Indiana. Lock your doors, send your fiancés to Europe, and cancel all buffet dinner parties.

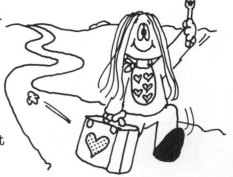

Not only do food and love march hand in hand, but a person's own particular relationship with food often exactly parallels her relationship with relationships.

Therefore, maybe if we could improve our relationship with food, we could improve our relationship with relationships.

Maybe we'll solve our food problems, fall madly in love, and live happily ever after.

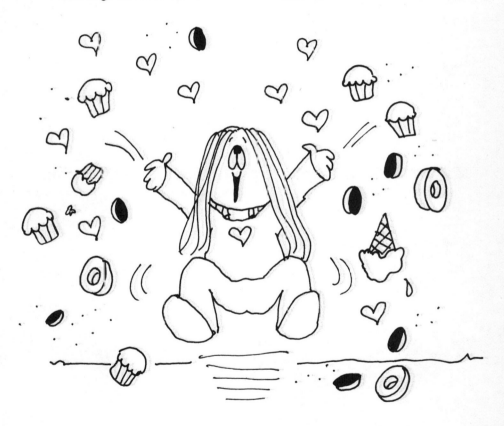

Maybe we'll all sprout wings and fly to the moon.

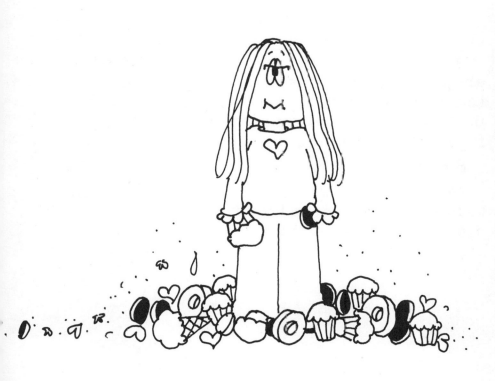

As long as the size 3 heroines in the movies
are going to go frolicking on the beach with
triple-dip ice cream cones and men who make
us drool, we are not going to drop that
food/love connection.

So forget it.

We must learn to manipulate our attachment
to food so it will work to our advantage in
dealing with relationships.

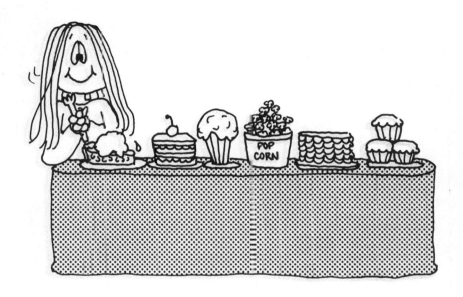

The following are six things to do with fattening food that will actually improve your relationships:

1. Order dessert as soon as you can
   in a relationship.

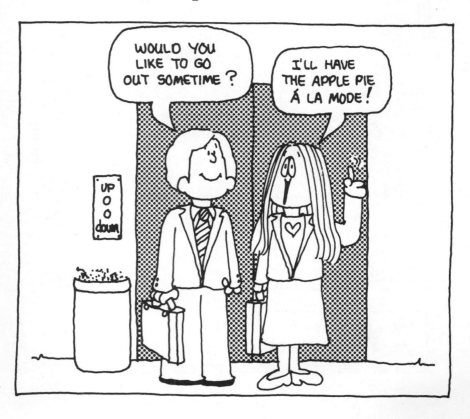

You can tell a lot about a man by how he reacts to you ordering a giant, fattening dessert.

If he says, "Do we really need that??" or starts telling you about his plump aunt who joined this really great weight loss group and lost seven pounds in three months, you will have some clue as to how much you may or may not want to invest in this particular relationship.

2. Eat your date's dessert.

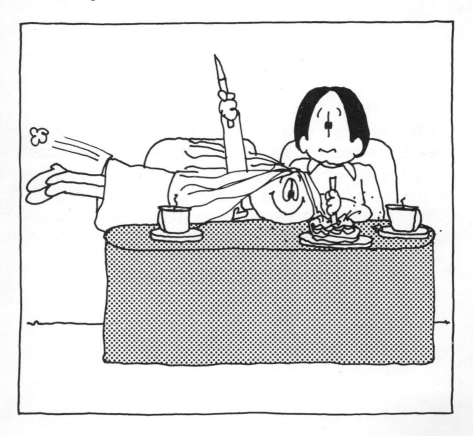

You can tell a lot about a man by how he reacts when you eat his entire dessert after swearing you didn't want any, not even a tiny taste.

Some men will shrug and chuckle and tell you you look beautiful when your cheeks are full of pineapple upside-down cake.

Some men will fling their bodies on their plates and not let you have any.

Some men will fling the incident in your face for the next six months.

"Remember that time you said you didn't want any dessert and you ate my entire pineapple upside-down cake?"

Bleah.

Better to find out early.

3. Eat chocolate when you're jealous.

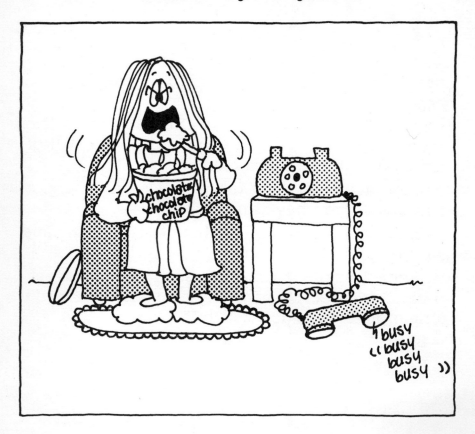

It is far better to eat a half-gallon of chocolate/chocolate chip ice cream than it is to charge over to your boyfriend's and break down the door, screaming, "AHAH! AHAH!" at 3:00 a.m.

It is easier to lose the weight you'll gain from a carton of Hostess Ho-Ho's, than it is to sabotage a mail truck, trying to retrieve a letter you wish you'd never sent.

When your suspicious little mind starts to bubble and brew with accusations, stop to consider: In the long run, which will you regret less? Eating 400 Milk Duds, or bursting into his office shrieking "I'VE GOT YOU NOW, YOU MISERABLE CHEAT!!!" at the top of your lungs?

4. Take your date to the movies and put him in charge of buying the refreshments.

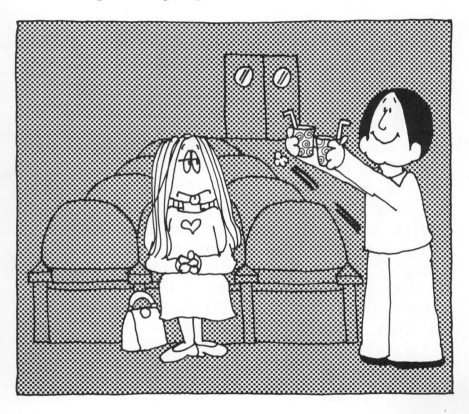

You can learn more about a man than a whole army of shrinks simply by noting what he thinks is an appropriate amount of food to buy for a two-hour movie.

The specific snacks he chooses, of course, are just as revealing.

The man who arrives at the seat you saved with two small sugar-free soft drinks is trouble.

The man who brings an armload of Milk Duds, Junior Mints, Goobers, Chuckles, Good'n 'Plenty's, Ice Cream Bon Bons, and a giant buttered popcorn . . . this man is worth considering.

Take him to more movies.

If by your sixth date he's deteriorated to, "Eh, we don't need anything to eat. I have some gum in my pocket" you'll know it's time to move on.

5. When your date is late, eat a Pepperidge Farm Cake.

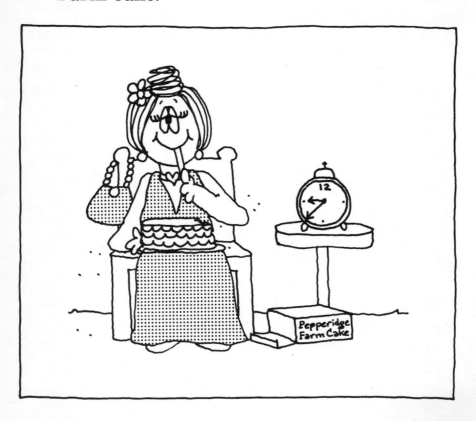

How many of us have torn home from the office, cleaned the entire house, hemmed and ironed an outfit, charged out to the store for new pantyhose, showered, shampooed, done our hair and makeup, and generally performed a total life makeover in one hour flat, only to have our dinner date wander in 45 minutes late?

Next time, eat a Pepperidge Farm Cake.

When he doesn't show up at five past the hour, take a Pepperidge Farm Cake out of the freezer and calmly start eating.

You won't get all sweaty pacing back and forth thinking up ways to murder him.

You won't ruin your hair by re-hot-rollering it 11 times.

You won't get a headache from composing vicious speeches.

And when he meanders up to the door and says "Hi. Ready for dinner?" you can smile and say with feeling, "Sorry, I already ate."

6. Make a cupcake be your alibi.

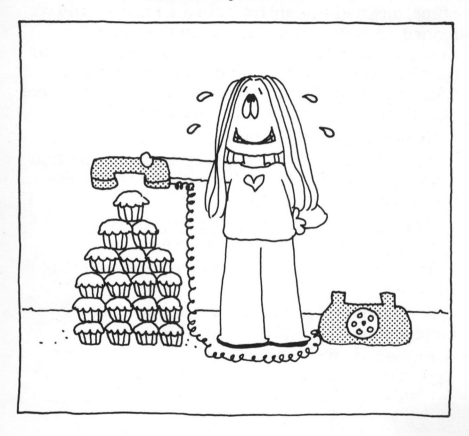

When you're lying on the living room floor trying to focus on "Fantasy Island" reruns and someone you don't want to go out with calls up and says, "Hi. Are you busy?" it's hard to say "Yes" and sound like you mean it.

If you have a plate of cupcakes lying there next to you, you never have to actually tell an outright lie. Hold a cupcake up to your mouth. "Yes. I'm busy."

I have to decide which cupcake to eat first. I have to decide whether to take the paper off first or just jump right in. I have to figure out how to position my mouth so I get some frosting on each and every bite. Then I have to eat the cupcakes. Then I have to clean up the mess. Then I have to go find more cupcakes. Busy, busy, busy.

"Yes. I am quite busy." The man will hang up. And you will suddenly feel quite grateful that you are on a date with a plate full of cupcakes.

"Oh, thank you, cupcake" . . .

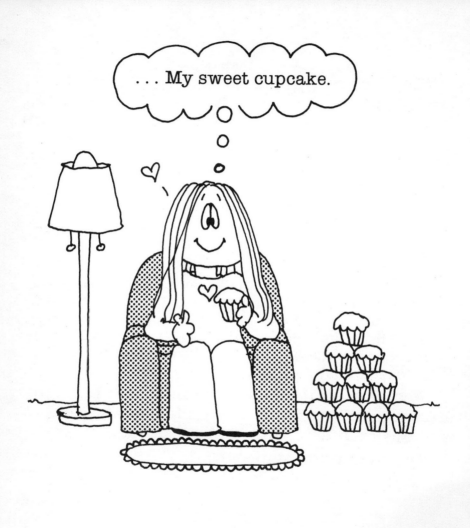

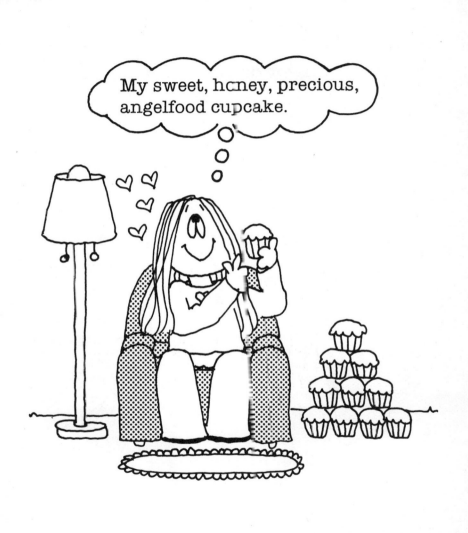

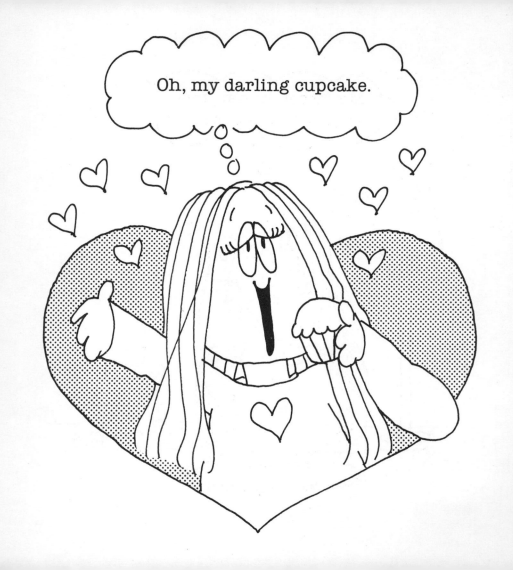

At least now we know how it all got started.